Florence Botto

An interior itinerary

Yoga

Florence BOTTO

An interior itinerary

Translated from French by Sara Stenhouse

Yoga

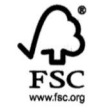

SUMMARY

ACKNOWLEDGEMENTS 7

FOREWORD 9

INTRODUCTION 11

    CHAPTER 1. THE PRINCIPALS OF TEACHING *YOGA* 13
    CHAPTER 2. THE BENEFITS OF *YOGA* 26
        1- *YOGA*, AN ODE TO NATURE 26
        2- *YOGA*, METAMORPHOSIS OF THE BODY'S EXPERIENCE 35
        3- *YOGA*, AN ELIXIR OF LONG LIFE 44
        4- *YOGA*, A PATH TO THE AWAKENING OF CONSCIOUSNESS 52

CONCLUSION 59

REFERENCES 61

GLOSSARY 65

© 2016 Florence BOTTO
Editeur BoD – Books on Demand
12/14 rond-point des Champs Elysées
75008 Paris
Impression BoD – Books on Demand, GmBH, Norderstedt
Allemagne

ISBN : 9 782322 011490

Dépôt légal : mai 2016

ACKNOWLEDGEMENTS

I would like to specially thank **Géraldine Dutruel** and **Amrita** for proof reading this manuscript.

FOREWORD

Let us observe with joy and emotion as often as possible the gift of life that constantly manifests itself in the three kingdoms of nature, so that our time on this planet may be a source of infinite inspiration.

Let us achieve strength of wisdom by creating harmony all around us and in all we do, in order to reveal with elegance the noblest aspect of our role as humans.

Let us explore, with the energy of *yoga*, the mystery of life; that part of the enigma may be unveiled to us: that we may meet our inner being and complete what remains of our existence.

INTRODUCTION

Just as the fate of our planet is bound by the behaviour of mankind, our own fate is bound by our attitude. Today, man is conscious that he holds the key to his well-being and that this key may be obtained through diligent practice of *yoga*. Now, more than ever, *yoga* has its place in our society.

***Yoga* as an exceptional heritage.**
To understand *yoga*, we need to look at its history and retrace its roots. *Yoga* is mentioned in many ancient fundamental texts, such as the Upanishads, the Bhagavad-Gita (which is one of the principal sections of the Mahabharata), and the Yoga-Sutras of Patanjali. References can also be found in the Gheranda Samhita, the Hatha Yoga Pradipika and the Shiva Samhita.

***Yoga* as a universal language.**
The discipline of *yoga* has become very popular with people of all ages, genders and occupation, regardless of belief, religion and nationality. The fact that interest is expected to continue to rise illustrates with striking intensity that this ancient practice passed down through the generations will never be lost.

***Yoga* as a benediction.**
Yoga is practiced with the body, the heart and the soul, as Yogananda explains: *"Yoga is an art as well as a science. It is a science, because it offers practical methods for controlling body and mind, thereby making deep meditation possible. And it is an art, for unless it is practiced intuitively and sensitively it will yield only superficial results."*[1]

A *yoga* class is a privileged moment during which we celebrate this sacred heritage and can benefit from its noble qualities. It is a journey in the vast universe of the inner Self and goes far beyond awareness of oneself, of others or of our surroundings: it is an invitation to respect, in the broadest sense of the word. It is a way of being.

CHAPTER 1. THE PRINCIPALS OF TEACHING *YOGA*

Teaching *yoga* is a privilege, and for a class to be perfectly measured, it must be planned with great care. For an instructor, *yoga* is an art that is practiced intensely in the knowledge that a session is constructed as the body is constructed. For the student (*sadhaka*), each lesson is a precious moment, a benediction that is welcomed with great willingness as it is not imposed and remains a personal choice. Each class is a moment entirely devoted to the Self, an adventure that goes beyond imagination.

A *yoga* session always has beneficial effects and results in a sense of well-being.

The following steps are important for maximum benefits:

1- **Prepare a class with intelligence.** To become a *yoga* instructor we need to live and breathe the spirit of *yoga*. This requires: 1) technical competence and persistent practice, 2) impartial assessment of training and discernment when it comes to comments that are read or heard. We cannot rely on simply informing participants of the risks and benefits of a posture without prior observation of effects on oneself and on our students. 3) Diligent and in-depth study of fundamental texts is also necessary.

2- **Be creative.** For learning to be a gentle and progressive experience for all, we must arrange the dynamics of a lesson by adapting instruction according to our students and their many differences (level of training, physical condition, motivation, any handicaps or illnesses.) Indeed, all participants (whether they are beginners or more advanced learners) cannot progress in one fell swoop, especially as each person will perceive the lesson differently according to his constitution, individuality, his favourite postures, his own manner of comprehending the session, etc. So, to be able to take into account each person's needs, the following steps will be helpful when planning, or even during a class.

- **Don't be afraid to mix *yoga* with other disciplines**, but take care not to popularize it. A good warm up for stiff joints will be appreciated by those who get little exercise during the week or may have experienced physical inactivity for some time.

- **Be flexible in your class planning and vary your approaches** to bring difficult postures within students' reach. Beware of over-zealous beginners; these students need help in measuring their efforts to avoid injury or over-exertion. For participants to get the very best from a class, propose several variants of postures and encourage them to choose and appropriate the posture they feel most comfortable in. It's important to note that the beginner *yogi* mustn't aim for a high technical level but rather a correct precision of postures, and take into account any physical boundaries they may have. This is why an instructor should open a class with variants of the simplest postures; it enables us to judge whether the basics have been correctly integrated. Pay particular attention to the position of the spine.

- **Use improvisation** as the best classes are those suggested by students. This means reducing the number of postures to respect each individual's rhythm; favour quality over quantity.

- **Aim for a method that can be used unassisted** to encourage practice outside class. This is advised in the two following cases: 1) when the rhythm of group sessions is elevated but a student still wishes to keep up and practice that style of *yoga*, 2) when keen learners are unable to attend regular group classes due to a busy lifestyle, but still want to practice daily.

3- **Reveal the rich complexity hidden by apparent simplicity.** Make sure that the basic structure of a lesson is coherent by:

- planning a natural flow from one posture to another with perceivable continuity throughout the class;

- explaining the posture or any other exercise that is being performed and providing additional thought to participants. A great deal of thought and reflection is required for a teacher to effectively employ his knowledge and experience to explain the advantages of a posture, an exercise or the lesson itself;

- going beyond the simple physical practice of *yoga*. Once students have mastered the technical aspect, the symbolic aspect and its recondite significance will follow naturally. This ultimately means focusing on the inner dynamic of a session: its strength.

4- **Avoid routine.**

- Particular attention has to be given to the organisation of a *yoga* lesson. To avoid the tedious traps of repetition throughout the year, take care to prioritize objectives and/or themes to create a natural flow. This isn't very hard as the possibilities are endless due to the abundance of tools available. Sequences become pleasant surprises and students experience and understand each class in a different way.

- However, remember that repetitive practice of certain poses in each class is required to encourage dedication to *yoga*. Improvement and consistence of practice extends and deepens knowledge of the soul and will attain and maintain oneness.

5- It hardly seems necessary to point out that **perfect knowledge of the anatomy and the physiology of the human body** isn't just an advantage but rather a pre-requisite.

A *yoga* class can be approached in multiple ways. No set plan can be produced and reproduced for a *yoga* lesson. Classes evolve according to the needs of our students and each lesson has its own specific nature and its own particular balance. It's only very progressively that the most subtle benefits of *yoga* will emerge. A clearer understanding can be had by sorting yoga's benefits into four chapters as described in this book, and then by explaining the specific assets of various elements that structure a lesson.

➢ **Raising awareness**

A *yoga* session starts with raising awareness through the dorsal decubitus position (for those with lower back problems advise the position with knees bent and feet on the floor). This brings awareness to each point of contact the body makes with the floor, consciousness of any tensions at the beginning of the session and a time of preparation for what will follow.

➢ Chanting sacred syllables or words or *mantras*

The Sanskrit word *mantra* consists of the root *man* (mind) and *tra* (tool); an instrument of thought. A *mantra* is a sequence of syllables, words or phrases chanted aloud or mentally. The art of continual repetition of *mantras* is called *japa* (a Sanskrit word meaning recitation).

Repeating a *mantra* is serenely allowing thoughts to unremittingly flow in and out of the mind, this can be with or without a *mala* (a rosary of 108 beads).

There are many *mantras* and each one has its own well defined intention or objective. One well-known *mantra* is *Aum* (or *Om*), considered Unique or Enduring or *ekakshara*, it is the root *mantra* or *mala mantra*, a primordial sound or *pranava*. It is hardly surprising that this syllable is placed above all other *mantras*.

➢ Sun salutation or *surya namaskara*

And so we come to the sun salutation. *Surya* is a Sanskrit term meaning sun and *namaskara* is Hindi and means salutation. This powerful workout awakens the body and warms its muscles, preparing it for the difficult stationary postures and various breathing exercises to come during the course of a lesson. The sun salutation is made up of two complete sequences (one for each side of the body), that consist of twelve *yoga* postures set to the respiratory rhythm. Taking into account each participant's physical condition will determine the even number of sun salutations to be performed.

Note that each posture can be associated with a *mantra*.[2]

- If the sun salutation is done at a fast pace we use the six following *bija mantras*:

    Posture 1 and posture 7: *Om Hram*.

    Posture 2 and posture 8: *Om Hrim*.

    Posture 3 and posture 9: *Om Hroom*.

    Posture 4 and posture 10: *Om Hraim*.

    Posture 5 and posture 11: *Om Hraum*.

    Posture 6 and posture 12: *Om Hraha*.

- If the sun salutation is done slowly we choose the following slower *mantras*:

    Posture 1: *Om Mitraya Namaha*.

    Posture 2: *Om Ravaye Namaha*.

    Posture 3: *Om Suryaya Namaha*.

    Posture 4: *Om Bhanave Namaha*.

Posture 5: *Om Khagaya Namaha.*

Posture 6: *Om Pushne Namaha.*

Posture 7: *Om Hiranya Garbhaya Namaha.*

Posture 8: *Om Marichaye Namaha.*

Posture 9: *Om Adityaya Namaha.*

Posture 10: *Om Savitre Namaha.*

Posture 11: *Om Arkaya Namaha.*

Posture 12: *Om Bhaskaraya Namaha.*

Surya Namaskara is best followed by a moment of rest in the dorsal decubitus position where cardiac and respiratory rates can return to normal. Participants can also soak up, reflect on and appreciate the wealth of sensations that follow the sun salutation.

> ### **Yoga postures or *asanas***

Asanas follow the sun salutation. The definition of *asana* is literally "to sit down", to adopt a sitting position.

Each posture consists of three stages; active (from entering the pose until leaving it), stationary (of variable length and intensity); and finally recovery. The range of postures has hardly changed since time immemorial, and decisive factors in the quality of a lesson are the abundance and incredible variety of both postures and instruction in *yoga*.

Each posture is specific and may be accompanied by:

- *mudras* (gestures and attitudes) that are particular to the positioning of the hands and arms,

- *bandhas* (literally meaning to seal) that are muscular contractions. There are three principal seals: the root seal (*mula bandha*), the upward flying seal (uddiyana bandha) and the throat seal (*jalandhara banha*). Note that we call the combination of *mula bandha, jalandhara banha* and *uddiyana bandha* the Great Lock (*mahabandha*), and mark it with a suspension of breath.

A few precious moments of reflection between poses in a relaxing position are as important as moving into or holding a posture, for any physical effort must be followed up by recovery which optimizes the effects of the pose. *Mantras* may be used to aid meditation.

> **Respiration and *pranayama* or breath control**

Breathing is a guide that emphasises fluidity in a *yoga* class. Like all catarrhines, man possesses nostrils that are close together and he will use them almost exclusively throughout a class as this is a natural reflex.

Generally, exercises of *pranayama* succeed a series of *asanas*.

The following steps distinguish:

- Exhalation (*rechaka*).

- Inhalation (*puraka*), which helps us to absorb the strength and quality of the energy acquired by calling upon our sense of perception and action (*indryas*).

- Retention (*kumbhaka*). This may be:
    - Either by holding the lungs full (*antara kumbhaka*), during which *prana* is held for a limited amount of time,
    - Or by holding the lungs empty (*bahya kumbhaka*).

When breath stops effortlessly this is a state of breath retention (*kevala khumbhaka*).

Breathing may also be associated with *mudras*.

➢ Concentration and meditation or *dharana* and *dhyana*

Concentration and meditation, with (or without) the use of *mudras*, enrich the range of discoveries and experiences that *yoga* has to offer. Because of this, it is possible to easily and comfortably hold any posture throughout this stationary journey, even if it lasts quite a long time.

The Mother, Mirra Alfassa, teaches us that concentration: *"... is to bring back all the scattered threads of consciousness to a single point, a single idea."*[3] In the same vein the Kshurika Upanishad, or the Cutting Knife Upanishad, explains: *"Who draws away the senses from the objects of sense* [manas], *as the tortoise draws in his limbs into the shell,* [pratyahara] *his intelligence sits firmly founded in wisdom."*[4]

Meditation is an implement that takes the *yogi* to a higher state of consciousness. Practice may be focused on visual objects such as light, say a flickering candle; or on a basic geometrical form known as a *yantra*. Meditation may also focus on the body by simply observing and experiencing the movements of the breath. *Mantras* may be used to aid meditation.

> **Final relaxation**

This is the recovery position that follows a *yoga* session. To bring an end to their adventure, students are invited to surrender themselves to gravity in a posture called the corpse pose (*shavasana*), the Sanskrit term *shav,* meaning corpse.

It is interesting to note that during the course of a *yoga* session it is possible to have brief encounters with life and death in all serenity.

CHAPTER 2. THE BENEFITS OF *YOGA*

1- *YOGA*, AN ODE TO NATURE

Human beings with all their preoccupations no longer connect with nature or gaze at the Universe with marvel, despite the fact that they constantly benefit from its generosity on all levels. Yet the Shiva Samhita teaches us: "*In this body, which is called Brahmanda (microcosm, literally the mundane egg), there is the nectar-rayed moon, in its proper place, on the top of the spinal cord...*"[5] To quote the Brahma Upanishad or Upanishad of the Brahman: "*A space, resembling a lotus-calyx, with its tip inclined downward, is the heart...*"[6]

Yoga classes are indeed a journey through space and time to the heart of nature that reveals the tight link that exists between man and the various kingdoms of nature. Indeed, they provide us with the opportunity to immerse ourselves in the kingdom of plant life. For example, when in the tree pose (*vrikshasana*), we can appreciate our verticality, an ancestral characteristic that we have shared with the world of plant life ever since the Australopithecus species acquired bipedalism over three million years ago. We can also reproduce poses and mime the behaviour of numerous animals, or we can blend into the mineral kingdom, notably by paying tribute to the sun (*surya*) and the moon (*chandra*). Moreover, according to the postures we perform, we can use thought to imagine different environments (terrestrial, aquatic, aerial) and thus experience their resulting atmospheres. The five elements, earth (*prithivi*), water (*jala*), fire (*agni*), air (*vayu*) and ether (*akasha*) are also implicitly present.

As a result, we become consciously aware that we represent a microcosm that is fully integrated into a macrocosm that together constitutes one and the same Universe. This act of immersion in nature is fundamental for the following reasons:

- **The Universe is saturated with rhythms**: the rhythm of the seasons, the precise movements of the stars, the alternating of day and night, the rhythm of tides, etc. As for the human being, the microcosm exists in the macrocosm and these are also animated, as aforementioned: the rhythm of the heart, the rhythm of breathing, the rhythm of thoughts, etc. The only problem is that twenty-first century man lives in incessant urgency, hence the advantages of regularly practicing *yoga* which slows down all our rhythms as a whole. This is most noticeable at the end of a class when a state of inactivity is particularly meaningful for the body, for the thoughts and for the emotions: it is a state of global inactivity of the Self.

- **Without energy there is no life** and any change needs the smallest amount of energy to be spent. Being bipedal is one of the characteristics of being humanoid and it represents a huge economy of energy compared to quadrupeds. These days, and in the context of the economic crisis that we are experiencing at present, our equilibrium, be it physical or mental, depends upon an ability to respond to unexpected and undesirable situations. The Universe produces the infinite vital energy (*prana*) that we need so much and it moves within the energy body (*pranamaya kosha*) and through veins and arteries (*nadis*). It penetrates our subtle energy centres (*chakras*) and when in a meditative state, ancient sages (*rishis*) likened them to lotus flowers where the number of petals symbolise the energy emitted from the *chakras*. There are six major *chakras* and all are linked to the *sushumna nadi*, which rises through the spinal cord and goes up to the top of the head, to the crown *chakra* (*sahasrara chakra*). Note that the distribution of *prana* in the body is controlled by the breath (*vayu*). *Yoga* is a medium we can apply to master the energy flow in the body; the practice of *yoga* draws on this powerful energy by means of the wealth of practices performed in a lesson. This may be breathing exercises, postures, sequences of poses, interiorizations, or any other exercise. For the body recharges itself with energy and stores it, but can also be freed from and thereby relieved of any excess energy.

➤ Chanting sacred syllables or words or *mantras*

A *mantra* is a vibration of sound set with energy and its conscious repetition enables this energy to be released. By using this procedure, its various rhythms gradually awaken the body. What's more, the Sanskrit language has intense emotional power and the simple act of hearing a *mantra* resonate or of hearing collective sounds made by other participants, can bring about a feeling of profound happiness and extreme well-being.

Of all *mantras*, *Om* is the symbol of supreme energy that serves the Universe.

➤ Sun salutation or *surya namaskara*

Dawn is the perfect time to celebrate this ancient method of respectful worship of sunrise. Thousands of years ago, the Ramayana poetically described this ritual:

Bend, Rama, bend thy heart and ear
The everlasting truth to hear
Which all thy hopes through life will bless
And crown thine arms with full success.
The rising sun with golden rays,
Light of the worlds, adore and praise:
The universal king, the lord
By hosts of heaven and fiends adored.
He tempers all with soft control,
He is the Gods' diviner soul;
And Gods above and fiends below
And men to him their safety owe.
He Brahmá, Vishu, Siva, he
Each person of the glorious Three,
Is every God whose praise we tell,
The King of Heaven, the Lord of Hell:
Each God revered from times of old,
The Lord of War, the King of Gold..."[7]

The rhythm with which we perform the sun salutation determines the effects on the body and it can be done at a fast pace to obtain a thorough physical warm-up, or at a slow pace for spiritual well-being. With practice it becomes obvious which method is best suited, but ultimately we simply need to surrender and allow the breath to guide us.

Before beginning *surya namaskara*, turn to face the sun, place hands together at the heart centre, allow your breathing to become effortless and gaze upon the gentle rays of the sun as they softly reach over the horizon. This preliminary step really helps us to experience the glorious colours that so well characterise this star.

While practicing the sun salutation, veneration of the sun is experienced with the entire being. Sometimes its strength may be felt, a surge of energy throughout the whole of the body, maybe even flowing into the heart. As the *asanas* are threaded together by the salutation, energy is gathered and dispersed, producing *prana*; and the more salutations we practice, the more we will perceive this flow of positive energy in the body.

At the end of a sun salutation, it's the peaceful pose of *shavasana* that allows us to appreciate the body's radiance.

> *Yoga* **postures or** *asanas*

The transition from sun salutation to *yoga* postures enables us to slow the physical and mental rhythms of our being. This also applies to the transition from an active stage to a stationary one.

What's more, each *yoga* posture generates its own energy and releases it throughout the whole of the body. Knowing this, we can easily understand that the choice of *asanas* that make up a class and their juxtaposition in a precise order represent a truly energetic fusion that will invigorate the soul. A brief pause between each posture helps to absorb the *prana* that's been generated.

Yoga brings contentment into our lives and by practicing with joy, happiness becomes a part of the inner being, thus giving us the energy we need to achieve our desires.

> **Respiration and** *pranayama* **or breath control**

Life is simply incessant macroscopic and microscopic breathing.

During a *yoga* session, breathing is our background music; throughout a class we can simply be aware of its natural rhythm, or change it by slowing it down or speeding it up. Breathing may be gentle or vigorous, shallow or deep, audible or barely perceptible, of so many different sounds...

Breathing brings an abundance of fresh new energy and the body takes what it needs and liberates the rest. Controlling the breath, or more importantly, lengthening each inhalation and each exhalation will increase the flow of *prana*.

By practicing different breathing techniques throughout a year of *yoga* sessions, students will really feel revitalized from these generous movements of *prana*.

> ➢ **Meditation or *dhyana***

A refreshing contact with nature really helps interiorization and the body is energized when concentration is directed towards nature. We can also progressively enter into a meditative state by simply being caught up by the rhythm of the breath. As a result, the body, thoughts and emotions are stilled, alpha wave activity is increased and the mind rests... utter bliss!

Meditation is also a source of energy. Before getting started, it's preferable to adopt a comfortable sitting position, keeping the spine perfectly straight so that energy may circulate freely. An intense process of interiorization is necessary;

this allows us to voluntarily guide and consciously absorb, then stock and distribute *prana* throughout the body. For example, directing attention towards a *chakra* by feeling its colour creates a vibrational state where energy is identical in colour to that of the *chakra* in question. So, just like a chameleon, the body takes on the characteristic hue of the different *chakras* and we really feel this vehicle of vivifying, animated and colourful sensations.

> **Relaxation**

As previously said, a rest between *yoga* postures helps us to absorb the *prana* that has been generated. The final relaxation is a strategic moment that indicates an important change in rhythm. Better control of the free flow of energy is all the more palpable, both on the surface as on other levels, and at this point relaxation is quite simply inner peace.

2- *YOGA*, METAMORPHOSIS OF THE BODY'S EXPERIENCE

Man has always wanted to control his environment, from what is infinitely small (as with the invention of the microscope) to what is infinitely large (as with the development of astronomical instruments and the telescope), but has he ever thought to observe himself with such clarity? This would mean internalizing awareness: on the one hand bearing with physical stillness and on the other hand struggling with the flood of thoughts that submerge him, all this subjecting the mind to projections of the past and the future.

In *yoga*, what is most important is living in the present. Once this has become a way of being we realize that everything communicates and exchanges on all levels.

- On Earth vegetation communicates with itself and with other species, insects for example.

- Mammals communicate in the same way by secreting hormones.

- The human body is also adept in the art of communication. Generally speaking, man perceives his body as an entity composed of organs, tissue and cells, without a face or name. *Yoga* reconciles us with our bodies so that we can appreciate the priceless wealth it represents. The *yoga* student has the opportunity to understand the body's many facets. This understanding develops the senses, even the most subtle senses, which help him master his thoughts.

We may wonder how *yoga* can bring this about so quickly.

- In modern society, vision is our main direct contact with the world. Man is endowed with a complex visual system and the significant development of the occipital lobe of the human brain bears witness to this. That being so, all simians have the ability to shut their eyes and when practicing *yoga* the eyelids are for the most part delicately closed over the eyes. This allows us to shut out the Universe and so avoids any distractions; progressively we slip from our outer bounds towards our inner being, and thereby merge with the Self. Our aim is to develop inner sight, refine listening skills and initiate inner dialogue.

- Everything around us in modern day life is noisy and even if *yoga* teaches us to disregard our immediate surroundings, it is impossible to escape them completely. What's more, some people are invaded by constant inner chatter that disturbs their daily life, which shifts their perception of reality and prevents awareness of their body language. This presents a real obstacle to attaining self-knowledge and self-realization, which is why inner silence (*antar mauna*) remains a priority throughout a class in order to free the mind of anything that is not part of the present. Patanjali referred to this conception *"If you can control the rising of the mind into ripples, you will experience Yoga."*[8] The Mother, Mirra Alfassa, further explains *"In fact, this is even the only way of establishing a constant silence in one's mind. It is to open oneself to higher regions and let this higher consciousness, force, light descend constantly into the lower mind and take possession of it."*[9] Stillness and silence allow us to truly let go (*vairagya*) and be led to a qualitative sensory perception, a prelude to the establishment of inner dialogue.

> ➤ **Chanting sacred syllables or words or *mantras***

There are three specific stages in repeating a *mantra*, first a vibration is made, then an inner resonance is felt and finally there is silence. The *mantra* represents a substitute to mental chatter, and is highly recommended as preparation for awareness.

➤ **Sun salutation or** *surya namaskara*

The sun salutation represents a search of an intense inner experience in the present moment with the sun as our guide.

With practice, it is also possible to concentrate on the *chakras* that are successively called upon by the different postures of *yoga*.

Further interiorization may be attained by reciting the *mantras* specific to each of the twelve postures that constitute the sun salutation.

Surya namaskara allows a *yogi* to become totally absorbed in this sequence of postures, which will imperceptibly lead him to inner silence, for it is in a founding silence that the sun salutation unfolds.

➤ *Yoga* **postures or** *asanas*

It is necessary to interiorize every instant while performing *asanas*, so that the posture is perfectly mastered and its maximum benefits are felt. The following instructions are a pleasant method.

1. Before entering a pose it is important to prepare it mentally. Imagine taking the posture, holding it and leaving it with ease. This visualization allows the pose to come naturally.

2. During the active stage, turn all attention to the technique of taking the posture and the flow of movements made, then make any necessary adjustments. This preparation will render a stationary pose easier and steadier rather than hamper it.

3. During the stationary stage, stay for as long as is comfortable by associating deep concentration, this helps to experience the posture through the muscles, the breathing and mentally too. Master thoughts with the following steps:

    - Be conscious of each movement that makes up the posture.

    - Observe how breathing adapts itself to each posture.

    - Guide thoughts to the areas that are most called upon to maintain the posture and relax the muscles accordingly.

- Accompany each inhalation and each exhalation with a mental *Om*.

- Adopt *Ujjayi* breathing, a word which means "to be victorious".

4. On leaving the pose, savour the benefits of an inner presence.

Having taken the steps above during the course of a posture, some people will feel a powerful flow of energy throughout body. If a silence progressively takes over the body, we know the posture has been mastered. This is when an inner dialogue has been established.

➢ Respiration and *pranayama* or breath control

The multitude of breathing and *pranayama* exercises proposed in *yoga* leave no room for distraction and this helps with the struggle against mental fluctuations. The Hatha Yoga Pradipika unveils an excellent attitude to have: *"All pranayama methods are to be done with a concentrated mind. The wise man should not let his mind be involved in the modifications (vrittis)."*[10] In the Yoga-Sutras of Patanjali, Sri Swami Satyananda quotes Patanjali and comments as follows: *"The modifications of the life-breath are either external, internal or stationary. They are to be regulated by space, time and number... According to Patanjali, there are three types of pranayama: the bahya vrtti, abhyantara vrtti and stambha vrtti - or inhaling, exhaling and retention... Place means where we place our attention while breathing: the base of the spine, its middle or higher regions, etc. Time means how long we retain our breath. Count refers to the amount of counts with which we take the breath in and with which we send it out and the number with which we hold it..."*[11]

The simple act of listening to respiration is an open window to the body in the present moment and observing respiration allows the senses to withdraw.

> ➢ **Concentration and meditation or *dharana* and *dhyana***

Concentration and meditation are also invitations to attain inner peace. The whole body lets go and becomes absorbed in the present. Persistent practice allows mental oscillations to be controlled.

Meditation is an excellent experience of silence, as Krishnamurti tells us: *"In meditation, which is to bring about a mind that is absolutely quiet, any form of effort is futile"*[12]. Therefore it is feasible to be in the presence of a true inner silence, if indeed that remains within reach; it is a silence that envelopes the whole body and consumes the entire Self. Antoine de Saint-Exupery felt this profound inner experience: *"I have always loved the desert. One sits down on a desert sand dune, sees nothing, hears nothing. Yet through the silence something throbs, and gleams..."*[13]

It is important to note that with intense practice, meditation can be done anytime and anywhere and even when surrounded by noise, as long as interiorization is attained.

➤ Recovery and relaxation

At the beginning of a session this growing awareness brings relief from nagging preoccupations and consciousness of the body as a whole; thereby we enter an inner world.

After practicing the sun salutation, between postures and after a breathing exercise or *pranayama*, it is important to relax the body, for this is when we are aware of any feelings that follow a pose. Many sensations can be felt: from heaviness to lightness, heat to cold, tension to relaxation, tingling located in different areas, awareness of the chakras, etc.

At the end of a class, relaxation brings about a state of well-being much more intense than that brought on by a period of recovery after a posture. This is when the ultimate benefits are felt; eyes may water, yawns and sighs are spontaneous. In short, a healing silence guides us to a new inner conversation.

3- *YOGA*, AN ELIXIR OF LONG LIFE

The human body has suffered many changes throughout evolution; mutations and successive transpositions during geological times have had an effect on the evolution of humans' genomes. What's more, during a lifetime the human body is subject to the three cosmic powers that are creation, conservation and destruction. Even if it proves itself to be extraordinarily adaptable, the body deserves care and attention. After all, what would be the point in long life if there wasn't that priceless happiness that we all know as good health? It's best to bear in mind that to have a body in good health, it is necessary to accept that illness is an upset of balance; it allows us to better know our body and to understand how it functions in order to detect any future imbalance and be able to act in accordance.

We owe it to ourselves to firstly make an effort to change for the better - this can be by mastering anger, excessive attachment or fear. Secondly, by paying attention to our thoughts, what we say and what we do, we can avoid hurting others and therefore avoid hurting ourselves. Having taken these steps and by practicing the wide panel of techniques available, the benefits of *yoga* can be felt on many different levels. The physical sensation of well-being is mirrored by a mental well-being as *yoga* restores the connection between the body and the mind, and as a consequence, maintains cohesion of the Self. This is partly why *yoga* preserves the healing powers of the body and represents a life-saving quality in a troubled world where the keywords are money, exploitation, indifference and deception.

Concurrently with practicing *yoga*, it is also necessary to have a healthy lifestyle. This means following the path of moderation, as Krishna taught Arjuna in the Bhagavad Gita: *"Verily this Yoga is not for him who eats too much or sleeps too much, even as it is not for him who gives up sleep and food, O Arjuna."*[14] In fact, and more particularly in the case of diet, it is best to consume fresh and well-balanced foods that will better nourish the vital constituents of the body (*dhatus*).

> ➢ **Chanting sacred syllables or words or *mantras***

Mantras enable *yoga* to conjugate itself with a liberated vocal device.

Mantras are largely in Sanskrit, the latter literally meaning "the perfect language", however the following alexandrine poem by Victor Hugo: *"O wisdom! O pure spirit! Supreme serenity!"*[15] is a *mantra* of the same magnitude. When chanting a *mantra* it is almost a matter of course that we find ourselves being gently rocked by its alchemy of sound, its nurturing waves propagating not only from cell to cell, but from thought to thought. Tension located in any part of the body is released, breathing becomes regular, the mind is calmed, subtle centres are cleansed and nurtured, and finally the whole being is revitalised as complete harmony is found.

> **Sun salutation or *surya namaskara***

There are a multitude of benefits to be had from practicing the sun salutation. Here are but a few:

- Healthy respiration comes about from synchronisation of the breath and physical movement. As a consequence blood is oxygenated; meaning the circulation of blood and *prana* is increased. What's more, the body heat that is produced (*tapas*) allows impurities to be burnt and any blocked *nadis* to be freed.

- Stimulation of the muscular system (as practically all muscles are used) and release of muscular tension. As the series of postures requires the coordination of several muscles, postural balance is optimised and coordination of movements made easier.

- Joint mobility is preserved.

- Suppleness is maintained, especially when bending and stretching the spine.

- Stamina is increased and resilience improved.

- Respiration, digestion and blood circulation are stimulated. Better blood circulation gives a radiant complexion and in fact, one dons many colours during the sun salutation, this is what restores glow to the skin.

- Stimulation of the nervous system.

- The refinement and elegance emanating from the body as a whole is translated into a new language founded on fluidity.

➤ Postures and gestures or *asanas* and *mudras*

Having taken care to align the body correctly, any postural work is done on all levels, whether it is forward or backward bends, extensions or inversions, twists or balancing poses. Throughout a session, postures (whether they be standing, sitting, lying on the back, the front or the side) are meshed together in order to mobilize each part of the body, each pose reinforcing the previous one. We can see that:

- suppleness and balance are obtained from practicing *asanas*;

- balancing postures, as their name indicates, develop physical balance and bring mental peace;

- inverted postures change inner attitude and so bring about union;

- certain postures purify the *nadis* so that energy can circulate freely.

When performing *asanas* the use of *mudras* enhances the benefits of *yoga*, *prana* is channelled and mental faculties are awakened.

Asanas can be complemented by the use of *bandhas*, which lift *prana* from lower centres to higher centres.

> ➢ **Respiration and *pranayama* or breath control**

A person under stress generally has shallow, irregular and erratic breath. *Yoga's* incredible palette of breathing techniques offers many benefits.
- It enhances oxygenation and carbon dioxide is better eliminated, which is particularly beneficial to those under stress.

- It relieves muscular tension in the main areas of the body, especially in the neck and shoulders.

- It has a calming effect on the mind when the volume of air inhaled and exhaled is equal.

- It improves digestion.

- It improves self-control so we can better relate to our environment on a daily basis, no matter what situation we find ourselves in (whether it is unexpected or even unsettling).

- It promotes recovery.

- It strengthens stamina.

In addition to breathing exercises, more advanced *yoga* students can try *pranayama*. Because it has an effect on the bodily humours (*doshas*), an experienced *yogi* will choose exercises accordingly. *Pranayama* is a key part of a *yoga* session as Patanjali reminds us: *"That [firm posture] being acquired, the movements of inhalation and exhalation should be controlled. This is pranayama."*[16] However, it is recommended to take care to purify and strengthen the body before practicing *pranayama* with long breath retentions.

The Hatha Yoga Pradipika warns: *"The correct balance of ... energy creates good health. Whenever these positive and negative flows are suppressed, blocked, dissipated or poorly distributed, disease inevitably results."*(17)

Bandhas used in conjunction with breathing techniques also help to better master energy flow.

➢ Concentration and meditation or *dharana* and *dhyana*

Concentration and meditation are regenerative getaways for the mind and body. Even if life seems on hold during their practice, palpable changes occur. When a person meditates they start to glow within a surprisingly short amount of time, even if this lapse of time is determined by their capacity to interiorize. The brain becomes uniquely receptive, and thereby enters a state of repose, the mind becomes calm, is soothed and neutral, and relaxation is both physical and mental, allowing energy to flow freely.

➢ Relaxation

According to the Hatha Yoga Pradipika: *"Lying flat on the ground with the face upwards, in the manner of a dead body, is shavasana. It removes tiredness and enables the mind (and the whole body) to relax."*[18] Indeed, a wave of well-being is released and engulfs the whole body, peace and serenity can be read on participants' faces as they experience profound tranquillity and a sense of refreshment.

A commentary by Swami Muktibodhananda under the guidance of Swami Satyananda Saraswati on verse 20, chapter 4 of the Hatha Yoga Pradipika describes what relaxation really is: *"Relaxation in yoga is a sattwic experience and not a tamasic one. Relaxation for a yogi ... it is a state of equipoise, balance and receptivity."*[19]

Learning to relax and let go is primordial throughout a *yoga* class, especially during relaxation. It provides the best conditions for somnolence which is vital for healthy balance, and gentle awakening allows us to leave a session with gratitude, feeling the full benefits it has had on the whole body.

4- *YOGA*, A PATH TO THE AWAKENING OF CONSCIOUSNESS

Yoga is a slow, inner development towards spiritual well-being. As a matter of fact, not only is *yoga* widely recognised by the wise and diligent for its benefits, but it is also the culmination of hard, persevering work for an accomplished yogi. It is about experiencing sacredness which in turn reveals *yoga's* more subtle benefits, namely connection with the inner Self.

But as we've seen in the previous chapters, a certain number of notions need to be assimilated to be able to reach this state of enlightenment.

- We need to understand that this amazing world that we live in is ruled by ignorance (*avidya*) and illusion (*maya*). It is only through hard, earnest work on oneself and with the help of *yoga*, that we can progressively avoid these traps.

- We need to set aside any negative intentions, thoughts, words or actions towards others. The Dalai-lama himself meditates daily on eight verses about thought transformation, as he explains:
  "When one whom I have benefitted with great hope
  Unreasonably hurts me very badly,
  I will learn to view that person

As an excellent spiritual guide."[20]

- We need to realize the advantages of closeness to nature; this consciousness allows us to see a divine light that is present all around us. This extract from the Bhagavad-Gita illustrates perfectly: *"The light of the sun that illumines all this world, that which is in the moon and in fire, that light know as from Me."*[21]

- We need to grasp the fundamental role of the body and, as long as inner chatter is silenced, it will reveal the inner light.

All the elements that make up a *yoga* class are extremely effective and they come together generously to open up a path of peace that leads to an inner space bathed in the light of Universal love.

> **Chanting sacred syllables or words or *mantras***

Mantras are pure benediction for the following reasons:
- They represent the process of creation: a sound is born, vibrates and is extinguished.

- They open a mysterious and secret window on the world of harmony for they each represent a most precious celestial concerto. A *mantra's* perfect tuning fills our very cells with light and thereby vibrates the soul.

- Singing a *mantra* and thinking of its meaning leads to freedom. This is the case of *Om*, which has to be the *mantra* par excellence, as described in the following extract from the Mandukya Upanishad or the Frog Upanishad: *"The word Om is the Imperishable; all this its manifestation. Past, present and future – everything is Om. Whatever transcends the three divisions of time, that too is Om."*[22] It isn't surprising that this *mantra* is well known as an elevating chant.

➢ **Sun salutation or *surya namaskara***

Dawn is when Brahma awakens so it is the most appropriate moment to practice a sun salutation. It embodies a spiritual dance that puts us into direct contact with the divinity hidden behind the star. This comparison of the sun and the divine appears clearly in the Mahabharata: *"...among lights and splendours I am the radiant sun..."*[23] In the same vein, the Taittiriya Upanishad says: *"He who lives in man, he who lives in the sun, are one."*[24], as does the Brihadaranyaka Upanishad: *"The sun is the honey of all beings; all beings the honey of the sun.*

The bright eternal Self that is in the sun, the bright eternal Self that lives in the eye, are one and the same; that is immortality, that is Spirit, that is all."[25] And so we open our hearts to delicious and divine energy.

When practicing a sun salutation we begin by lifting attention to the sky in order to meet with the star. This is a way to reach the sun of the microcosm which enlightens the body and mind and with practice, the soul is bathed in light. Thus, we experience the following words of Sri Satyananda Saraswati: *"Developing practice of surya namaskara can have repercussions on our whole lifestyle and attitude to life. The exploration of ourselves that we initiate in our daily practice expands in concentric circles out into our daily activity, movement, interaction with people and things and thus helps to change our lives in a positive and creative way."*[26]

➢ Postures and gestures or *asanas* and *mudras*

Over years of practice, the symbolism of postures is experienced intensely, and like the stars in the sky they will fill the body with light and awaken consciousness. When postures are associated with *mudras*, awareness is further broadened.

➤ Respiration and *pranayama* or breath control

Breathing is a primordial function of the body in more than one way; it makes us conscious of a unity that represents our microcosm in which everything is bound together, each element or function influences another. B.K.S Iyengar explains this perfectly in his book Light on Pranayama: *"The purpose of pranayama is to make the respiratory system function at its best. This automatically improves the circulatory system, without which the processes of digestion and elimination would suffer. Toxins would accumulate, diseases spread through the body and ill-health becomes habitual. The respiratory system is the gateway to purifying the body, mind and intellect. The key to this is pranayama."*[27]

What's more, it should be noted that subtle energy (*prana*), binds all things in the Universe. With each respiration that fills the body with *prana*, a breath of freedom is brought into an enlightened space deep within. It is with this stillness of the body that thoughts and emotions are borne by breathing and some will perceive an energy that comes from the macrocosm and illuminates the microcosm. Finally, we can read in the Dhyana Bindu Upanishad: *"Brahma is said to be inspiration; Vishnu is said to be cessation (of breath) and Rudra is said to be expiration. These are the devatas of pranayama."*[28], and similarly Kabir writes: *"God is the breath of all breath."*[29]

Inspired by such wisdom, our breathing has a taste of total communion with the divine, a real privilege!

➢ Meditation or dhyana

According to Gheranda Samhita: *"There are said to be three types of dhyan: gross, luminous, and subtle. Gross is of an image and luminous is of light. Subtle dhyana is of bindu. It is Brahman, and Kundalini is the ultimate deity"*[30]

Meditation will satisfy any daring adventurer, for these inner explorations show us that the Self doesn't correspond with this limited space that we know: we can attain different states of consciousness that allow us to reach far horizons, and even cross the barrier of time. Meditation is a synchronisation of the Self, a surprising sensation of going back to the beginning, to *the* beginning...in other words, it is ultimate freedom!

➢ Relaxation

This inner experience, born of the efforts made throughout a session, brings us quite peacefully to a realization based on the oscillations of different levels of consciousness, be they spatial or temporal. We feel a spiritual freedom. Those who are comfortably in touch with their inner selves may even feel the Universal Spirit. This is how the mystery of the Self is revealed and as a result, the inner Self can rest.

CONCLUSION

The experience of *yoga* is a gift of life that changes the course of our existence. In the same manner of an alchemical transformation, Paulo Coelho writes: *"So that everyone will search for his treasure, find it, and then want to be better than he was in his former life."*[31]

The more we practice with regularity and enthusiasm, the more its wealth is unveiled. The inner Self is illuminated from within, becomes nurtured by wisdom and respect, and the worth of others becomes apparent, as evidenced in the book The Prophet: *"It is in the vast man that you are vast, And in beholding him that I beheld you and loved you."*[32]

Yoga has to be really lived. If we want to be able to understand what *yoga* fundamentally is and hope to experience an authentic transformation, persistent practice is necessary. We become the alchemist of the inner Self by gathering postures, breathing exercises or any other exercise according to the requirements of the present moment. We then appreciate steady inner-growth, feelings of humility and gratitude for the forces of nature that regulate the human body, and on a larger scale, life on Earth and in the Universe as a whole. Finally, we can approach life with enough dignity and confidence to be able to cope with the difficulties that we face and attempt to take the honourable path.

Man's greatest conquest is himself, and we have it within our grasp to be aware of this and experience it through *yoga*. So don't wait, and if you really wish to, live that great adventure called *yoga* from now on.

"I meditate upon the splendour of the Supreme Being, who with a sole breath created an infinity of worlds.
May its brilliant rays bring light to the very core of my soul, may it lead me from darkness to light, from ignorance to knowledge, and from death to immortality.
May this be so for all beings, from the smallest atom to the entire galaxy.
AUM"[33]

Let these words from the Gayatri *mantra* blossom deep within us and guide us towards pure light.

REFERENCES

(1)	The Essence of Self Realization. The Wisdom of Paramhansa Yogananda. Recorded and compiled by his disciple Swami Kriyananda (J.Donald Walters). Crystal Clarity Publishers 1990.
(2) (26)	Surya Namaskara (A Technique of Solar Vitalization) by Swami Satyananda Saraswati. Published by the Bihar School of Yoga, Munger, Bihar, India, 1983.
(3) (9)	The Sunlit Path, passages from conversations and writings of The Mother (Mirra Alfassa). Published by the Sri Aurobindo Ashram Publication Department, 2012.
(4) (14) (21) (23)	Bhagavad Gita and its Message by Sri Aurobindo, edited by Anilbaran Roy. Published by the Sri Aurobindo Trust, Pondichery, India, 1995.
(5)	The Siva Samhita. Translated by Rai Bahadur Srisa Chandra Vasu. Published by The Pânini Office, Bhuyaneswari Asrama, Bahadurganj, 1914.

(6)	Sixty Upanishads of the Veda, Volume II by Paul Deussen. Motilal Banarsidass Publishers Private Limited, 2004.
(7)	The Ramayan of Valmiki. Translated into English Verse by Ralph T. H. Griffith, M.A., Principal of the Benares College. Published by Truebner & Company, 1870-1874.
(8) (11) (16)	The Yoga-Sutras of Patañjali. Translation in English and commentary by Sri Swami Satchidananda. Integral Yoga Publications, revised edition 2012.
(10) (17) (18) (19)	Hatha Yoga Pradipika. Commentary by Swami Muktibodhananda under the guidance of Swami Satyananda Saraswati. Published by Yoga Publications Trust, Munger, Bihar, India, 2006.
(12)	This Light in Oneself, True Meditation by J. Krishnamurti. Published by Krishnamurti Foundation Ltd. 1999.
(13)	The Little Prince by Antoine de Saint-Exupery. Published by Mammoth, an imprint of Reed Books Limited, 1991.

(15)	Translated from Les Rayons et Les Ombres XLIV. Sagesse - A Mademoiselle Louise B by Victor Hugo. Published by Société d'Editions Littéraires et Artistiques, Paris. 1925.
(20)	The Union of Great Bliss and Emptiness. Teachings on the Practice of Guru Yoga by The Dalai Lama, translated by Geshe Thupten Jinpa. Snow Lion Publications, 1988.
(22) (25)	The Ten Principal Upanishads, put into English by Shri Purohot Swami and W.B. Yeats. Published by Faber and Faber Limited, 1952.
(24)	Upanishad Series N°7. Taittiriya-Upanishad by Swami Sharyananda. Published by The Ramakrishna Math, 1921.
(27)	Light on Prāṇāyāma, PranayamaDīpikā by B.K.S. Iyengar, and introduction by Yehudi Menuhin. The Aquarian Press, an imprint of Harper Collins Publishers, 1992.
(28)	Thirty Minor Upanishads by Narayanasvami Aiyar. Madras, printed by Annie Besant at the Vasanta Press, 1914.

(29)	The Songs of Kabir translated by Rabindranath Tagore, introduction by Evelyn Underhill. Published by The Macmillan Company, 1915.
(30)	The Gheranda Samhita. The Original Samskrit and An English translation by James Mallinson. Published by Yoga Vidya, 2004.
(31)	The Alchemist by Paulo Coelho. Published by Harper Collins Publishers, 1992.
(32)	The Prophet by Kahlil Gibran. Published by Penguin Books, 1998.
(33)	Translated from Yoga Polaire by François Brousse. Published by Editions La Licorne Ailée, 2012.

GLOSSARY

Please find below the transliteration in Roman script, the pronunciation of Sanskrit is enclosed in square brackets.

A

Agni: fire, one of the five elements.

Akasha [Ākāśa]: ether or space, one of the five elements.

Antar mauna: inner silence.

Arjuna: a principal character from the Bhagavad-Gita [*Bhagavad-Gītā*].

Asana [Āsana]: a yoga posture. Third stage of Patanjali's eightfold yoga [Patañjali].

Aum [Auṃ]: see *Om* [*Oṃ*].

Avidya [Avidyā]: ignorance.

B

Bandha: binding or capturing which involves contraction of certain muscles or parts of the body.

Bhagavad-Gita [Bhagavad-Gītā]: meaning the Divine Song. A Hindu saga from the Mahabharata [*Mahābhārata*] relating dialogues between Krishna [*Kṛṣṇa*] and Arjuna.

Bija mantra [Bīja mantra]: *bija* means seed, a powerful and generally monosyllabic mantra.

Bindu: a point.

Brahma [Brahmā]: one of the gods of the Hindu triad, the concept of creation.

Brahman: the Supreme Being.

C

Chakra [Cakra]: a wheel, a centre of energy also called *padma* or lotus. *Chakras* are located in the subtle body. There are seven principal energy centres, classed from the base of the chest to crown of the head.

- *Muladhara chakra [Mūlādhāra cakra].*
- *Swadhishthana chakra [Svādhiṣṭhāna cakra].*
- *Manipura chakra [Maṇipūra cakra].*
- *Anahata chakra [Anāhata cakra].*
- *Vishudda Chakra [Viśuddha cakra].*
- *Ajna chakra [Ājñā cakra].*
- *Sahasrara chakra [Sahasrāra cakra].*

Chandra [candra]: the moon.

D

Dharana [Dhāraṇā]: mental concentration. Sixth stage of Patanjali's eightfold yoga [Patañjali].

Dhatus [Dhātus]: constituents of the body.

Dhyana [Dhyāna]: Meditation. Seventh stage of Patanjali's eightfold yoga [Patañjali].

Dosha [Doṣa]: a mood or bodily humour. There are three types of *dosha*.

- *Vāta,* the dominating elements being ether and air.
- *Pitta,* the dominating elements being fire and earth.
- *Kapha,* the dominating elements being earth and water.

G

Gheranda Samhita [Gheraṇḍa Saṃhitā]: a classic text on Hatha Yoga [Haṭha Yoga] compiled by the the sage Gheranda *[Gheraṇḍa]*.

Gunas [Guṇa]: fundamental qualities of nature.
- ***Rajas:*** This represents movement, activity based on desires, attachment or passion.
  Rajasic: characterised by the qualities of rajas.
- ***Sattva:*** This represents balance, purity, wisdom, harmony.
  Sattvic: characterised by the qualities of *sattva*.
- ***Tamas:*** This represents the unconscious, inertia.
  Tamasic: characterised by the qualities of *tamas*.

H

Hatha Yoga Pradipika: a classic text on Hatha Yoga (the yoga of postures) compiled by Svatmarama [Svātmārāma].

I

Indriya: an organ of the senses.
- ***Jnanendriya [Jñānendriya]:*** the five organs of perception, namely the ears, the skin, the eyes, the tongue and the nose.
- ***Karmendriya:*** the five organs of action, specifically the voice, the hands, the feet, the anus and the genitals.

J

Jala: water, one of the five elements.

Jalandhara bandha [Jālandhara bandha]: the seal of the throat corresponds with a contraction of the throat. The energy centre implicated is *vishuddha chakra*.

Japa: continuous repetition of a *mantra*.

K

Kosha [Kośa]: a sheath. The human being is made up of the following five sheaths (from the most subtle to the least subtle).

- ***Anandamaya kosha [Ānandamayakośa]:*** the sheath of bliss.
- ***Vijnanamaya kosha [Vijñānamayakośa]:*** the sheath of intellect, of higher understanding.
- ***Manomaya kosha [Manomayakośa]:*** the sheath of the mental awareness.
- ***Pranamaya kosha [Prāṇamayakośa]:*** the sheath of vital energy.
- ***Annamaya kosha [Annamayakośa]:*** the sheath of food.

Krishna [Kṛṣṇa]: the eighth incarnation of Vishnu. He instructs Arjuna in yoga in the Bhagavad-Gita [*Bhagavad-Gitā*].

Kumbhaka: the suspension of breath.

- ***Antara kumbhaka:*** suspension of breath with lungs full.
- ***Bahya kumbhaka:*** suspension of breath with lungs empty.
- ***Kevala kumbhaka:*** natural cessation of breath.

Kundalini [Kuṇḍalinī]: the potential energy lying dormant in the human being and nestled in the *muladhara chakra [Mūlādhāra cakra]*.

M

Mahabandha [Mahābandha]: the great lock is the combination of all three *bandhas* (*mula bandha [mūla bandha], jalandhara bandha [jālandhara bandha]* and *uddiyana bandha [uḍḍiyāna bandha]*.

Mahabharata [Mahābhārata]: an epic poem of ancient India which includes the Bhagavad-Gita [*Bhagavad_Gītā*], authorship is attributed to Vyasa [*Vyāsa*].

Mala [Mālā]: a rosary of 108 beads.

Manas: the mind.

Mantra: chanted sacred syllables or words.

Maya [Māyā]: illusion.

Mudra [Mudrā]: gestures and postures used in conjunction with breathing exercises to lock and guide cosmic energy flow throughout the body and the mind.

Mula bandha [Mūla bandha]: the root lock, a contraction of the muscles of the perineum. Its corresponding energy centre is the muladhara chakra [*Mūlādhāra cakra*].

N

Nadi [Nāḍī]: a vein, artery or channel. There are many subtle channels in the body in which energy flows. There are three principal *nadis*.

- ***Ida nadi [iḍā nāḍī]*** in which lunar energy flows.
- ***Pingala nadi [piṅgalā nāḍī]*** in which solar energy flows.
- ***Sushamna nadi [suṣumṇā nāḍī]*** which is the main channel of energy.

Namaskara: a greeting or offering of respect.

O

Om [Oṃ]: a sacred monosyllable which is the Brahman of sound.

P

Panchamahabhuta [Panchamahābhuta]: the five elements – earth (*prithivi*), water (*jala*), fire (*agni*), air (*vayu*) and ether (*akasha*).

Prana [Prāna]: vital energy or life-force.

Pranamaya kosha [Prāṇāyāma]: see *kosha* [Kośa].

Pranava [Praṇava]: the primordial *mantra*.

Pranayama [Prāṇāyāma]: control and mastery of the breath. Fourth stage of Patanjali's eightfold yoga [Patañjali].

Pratyahara [Prayāhāra]: the mastering of the senses. Fifth stage of Patanjali's eightfold yoga [Patañjali].

Prithivi [Pṛthivī]: earth, one of the five elements.

Puraka [Pūraka]: inhalation.

R

Ramayana [Rāmāyaṇa]: an epic poem relating the life of Rama (seventh incarnation of Vishnu). Authorship is ascribed to the Hindu sage Valmiki [Vālmīki].

Rechaka [Recaka]: exhalation.

Rishi [Ṛṣi]: a seer, an illumined sage.

Rudra: epithet of Shiva, he is the destroyer of existence.

S

Sahaka [Sādhaka]: a spiritual aspirant who practices the discipline of yoga in order to achieve self-realization and spiritual consciousness.

Sarasvati [Sárasvatī nadī]: mystical flowing waters.

Sattvic: see *Gunas*.

Shavasana [Śavāsana]: posture of relaxation, the corpse pose.

Shiva Samhita [Shiva saṃhitā] or Siva Samhita [Siva saṃhitā]: a classic text on Hatha Yoga [Haṭha Yoga].

Surya [Sūrya]: the sun.

Sushumna nadi [suṣumṇā nāḍī]: one of three principal channels.

Swami [Svāmi]: a teacher or master of transcendental knowledge and self-realization who is freed of his senses.

U

Uddiyana bandha [Uḍḍiyāna bandha]: the upward flying lock. The abdominal muscles are forcefully contracted and pulled up towards the diaphragm. The energy centre for this *bandha* is the *manipura chakra [maṇipūra cakra]*.

Ujjayi [Ujjāyi]: *pranayama* is employed by slightly contracting the epiglottis which creates a vibrating sound.

Upanishad [Upaniṣad]: word suggesting the act of sitting at the feet of a master to receive his instruction.

V

Vairagya [Vairāgya]: a state of detachment, impassivity.

Vayu [Vāyu]: air, one of the five elements. There are five vital airs or currents.
- ***Prana vayu [Prāna vāyu]:*** the vital ascending energy of breathing.
- ***Apana vayu [Apāna vāyu]:*** the vital descending energy of breathing.
- ***Samana vayu [Samāna vāyu]:*** the vital energy of digestion and assimilation.
- ***Udana vayu [Udāna vāyu]:*** the vital energy of expression.
- ***Vyana vayu [Vyāna vāyu]:*** the vital energy that emanates from the centre of the body.

Vishnu [Viṣṇū]: one of the gods of the Hindu triad, the concept of preservation and protection.

Vrikshasana [Vrkāsana]: the tree pose.

Vritti [Vṛtti]: thought fluctuations, mental agitation.

Y

Yantra: a geometrical form.

Yoga: coming from the Sanskrit root *yug* meaning to join together but also to attach or direct attention to the mind. *Yoga* is union with the Self.

Yoga-Sutra [Yoga sūtra]: a compilation of 196 aphorisms on *yoga* by Patanjali [Patañjali].

Yogi [Yogī]: refers to a male practitioner of *yoga*. Note that a ***Yogini [Yoginī]*** denotes a female practitioner of *yoga*.